I0407933

The Food Cop™
NUTRITION GUIDE
and WORKBOOK

Second Edition

This book belongs to

_____

The Food Cop™
NUTRITION GUIDE
and WORKBOOK

Your Personal Resource for Healthy Eating

Second Edition

By Corinne Kantor, BS, DTR, CLT

The Food Cop: Nutrition Guide and Workbook. Copyright © 2017 by Corinne Kantor. Published by The Food Cop in the United States of America. All rights reserved. No other part of this book may be reproduced in any form or by any electronic or mechanical means, including information storage and retrieval systems, without permission in writing from the author, except by a reviewer, who may quote brief passages in a review. For more information, please contact The Food Cop, www.thefoodcop.com, info@thefoodcop.com.

Although the author and publisher have made every effort to ensure the accuracy and completeness of information contained in this book, we assume no responsibility for errors, inaccuracies, omissions, or any inconsistency herein. Any slights of people, places, or organizations are unintentional. The author disclaims any liability arising directly or indirectly from the use of this book.

First edition 2011
Second edition 2017

All trademarks are the property of their respective owners.

ISBN-13: 978-1544071411
ISBN-10: 1544071418

To receive an electronic newsletter containing information about nutrition and The Food Cop's upcoming events, visit www.thefoodcop.com.

ATTENTION CORPORATIONS, UNIVERSITIES, COLLEGES, AND PROFESSIONAL ORGANIZATIONS: Quantity discounts are available on bulk purchases of this book for educational, gift purposes, or as premiums for increasing magazine subscriptions or renewals. Special books or book excerpts can also be created to fit specific needs. For more information, please contact The Food Cop, www.thefoodcop.com, info@thefoodcop.com.

Photography by John Cordes.

Contents

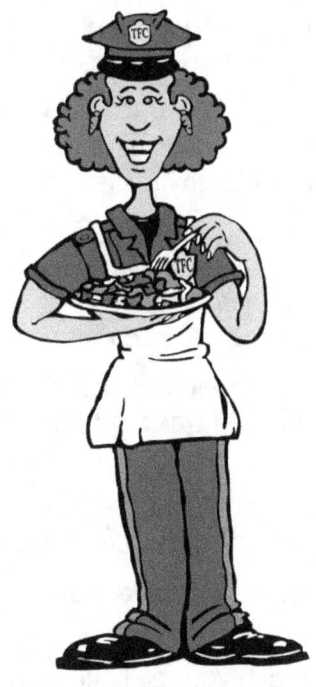

Welcome

ABOUT THIS BOOK

Congratulations on making the decision to live a healthier lifestyle! With the proper nutrition and exercise habits, you will be taking the necessary steps towards being a healthier you!

This book is designed to educate you in basic nutrition and provide you with a simple way to keep track of your nutrition consumption.

The first part of this book (Nutrition Guide) contains general nutrition information to help you make healthy decisions regarding your meal choices.

The second part of this book (Vitamin & Mineral Guide) contains information about fat-soluble and water-soluble vitamins, minerals, and the recommended food sources for each.

> Before starting any nutrition management or exercise regimen, be sure to consult with your physician.

The third part of this book (Workbook) allows you to keep track of your daily meal and nutrient intake — studies suggest that people who keep track of this information are more successful in achieving their goals.

This book also contains a section to make notes and post photos about your progress, along with a recommended serving size pocket guide that you can cut out and keep with you at all times.

Keep in mind that individual nutrition needs vary and are based on various factors, including age, sex, and health status.

Let's begin by taking a quiz to see how much you really know about healthy eating.

1. Which of the following is considered to be a "good" type of fat?
    *   Hydrogenated oil
    *   Monounsaturated and polyunsaturated fat
    *   Trans fat and saturated fat

2. Which of the following is true about nuts?
    *   Fattening no matter what
    *   High-calorie but good for you in small doses
    *   Mostly full of trans fats

3. Low-carbohydrate diets can put you at risk for
    *   Insufficient nutrients
    *   Gaining weight
    *   Osteoporosis

4. Peas and beans are good plant sources of
    *   Protein
    *   Monounsaturated fat
    *   Cholesterol

5. Which of the following is a primary risk factor for diabetes?
    - A high-sugar diet
    - A low-carbohydrate diet
    - A high-calorie diet

6. Skipping breakfast is a good way to
    - Gain weight
    - Curb your appetite later in the day
    - Lose weight

7. Which of the following are lean meats?
    - T-bone steak, pork chop, hamburger
    - Sausage, bacon, hot dog
    - Chicken breast, tuna, pork tenderloin
    - Cheese, goose, meatloaf

8. When deciding whether to eat a certain food item, you should
    - Decide if it is good or bad for you
    - Learn how it can reduce the chance of illness
    - Determine its appropriate role in the context of all other food choices

9. Potatoes and corn are considered to be
    - Vegetables
    - Meat
    - Starches

10. A nutrition label states that a food product contains green beans, carrots, red pepper, milk, and salt. Which of these ingredients is present in the highest quantity?
    - Salt
    - Green beans
    - Red pepper

11. The most effective way to reduce fat intake is to
    - Eliminate fats used as seasonings
    - Consume fewer snacks during the day
    - Replace butter with margarine

12. High protein diets are associated with
    - High fat foods
    - Improved kidney function
    - Decreased risk of heart disease

13. The best way to control salt intake is to
    - Control use of salt shakers
    - Stop using instant food
    - Limit intake of processed and fast food

14. Which of the following is directly associated with risk of heart disease?
 • Total cholesterol
 • HDL cholesterol
 • LDL cholesterol

The answers are on page 51.

GOALS AND OBSTACLES

When making a lifestyle change, it is important to set goals — realistic long-term and short-term goals that are manageable and attainable. Unrealistic goals might make you feel discouraged and could set you up for failure.

> Feeling discouraged? Don't give up! Review your goals to make sure they are realistic and attainable!

Short-term goals serve as "baby steps" in helping you achieve your long-term goals. For example, if your long-term goal is to decrease the amount of sweets you eat, you could begin by choosing frozen yogurt instead of ice cream on one day, and then another day, choose healthier toppings, such as nuts instead of chocolate chips, in addition to the frozen yogurt.

Goals should also be specific so you can see your progress. For example, if your long-term goal is to decrease your body fat percentage, you can check your body fat on a weekly or monthly basis. Use the workbook section in this book to keep track of your body fat percentage.

Unfortunately, obstacles may come up that get in the way of your progress. You must also determine the best way to deal with these obstacles. For example, while on vacation and eating out often, how can you watch your intake of foods high in saturated fat? During the holidays, how can you minimize your intake of sweets?

Take some time to write down your long-term goals, along with some short-term goals that will help you achieve these long-term goals.

GOALS

Long-Term Goal:	
Short-Term Goals:	

Long-Term Goal:	
Short-Term Goals:	

Long-Term Goal:	
Short-Term Goals:	

Long-Term Goal:	
Short-Term Goals:	

Long-Term Goal:	
Short-Term Goals:	

Long-Term Goal:	
Short-Term Goals:	

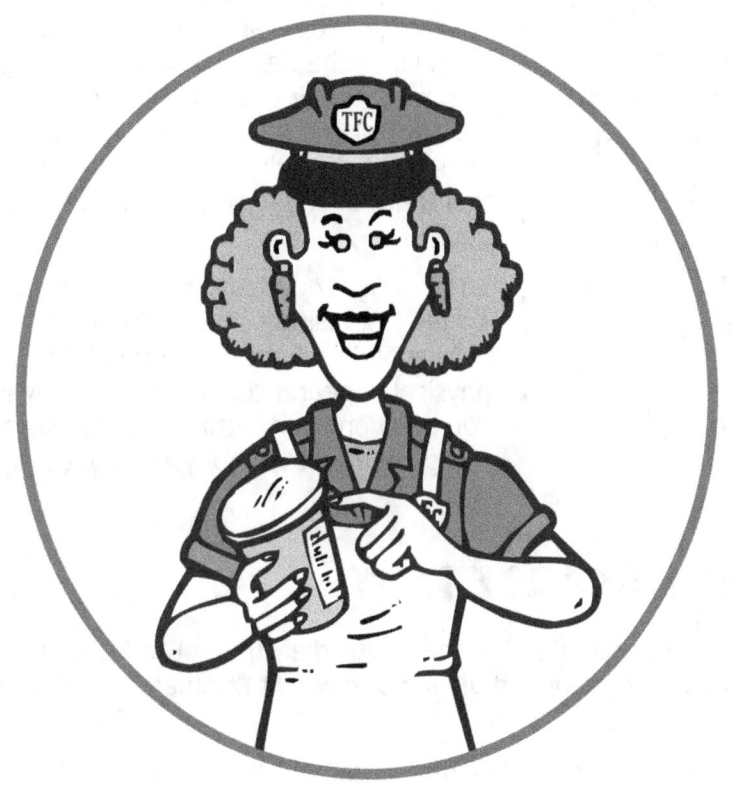

Nutrition Guide

This section contains general nutrition information to help you make healthy meal choices.

DIET VS. A HEALTHY LIFESTYLE

Diet: "to select or limit the food one eats to improve one's physical condition or to lose weight"

Lifestyle: "a manner of living that reflects the person's values and attitudes"

> Many people skip breakfast because they want to sleep in or they are not hungry. However, when you sleep, you lose energy. Breakfast is important because it gives you the energy you need to start your day.

Most people go on diets to lose weight, and they do this by temporarily changing the amount and type of food they eat. Some people also choose to start an exercise regimen. Once the desired amount of weight has been lost, they go off their diet and back to their normal eating habits. They also tend to stop exercising. Sometimes people give up on their diet and losing weight, and go back to their normal eating habits without reaching their desired goal.

Living a healthy lifestyle is a lifelong commitment. It is not simply just losing or managing your weight temporarily to reduce and prevent health problems and improve your physical appearance. Living a healthy lifestyle can make you emotionally healthier and happier as well — when you feel good about your physical appearance, it helps you feel better inside.

DEBUNKING FAD DIETS

The Cabbage Soup diet, the Chocolate diet, the Atkins diet, the South Beach diet, the Grapefruit diet...these are just some of the many fad diets that have hit the market and we have experimented with over the years.

Their claims sound great — quick, easy weight loss without much exercise involved, if any, and you can be thin for the rest of your life.

However, what many people don't realize is how dangerous these diets can be, both physically and psychologically. Many fad diets tend to over-emphasize one particular food item, or type of food, which contradicts the guidelines for healthy eating. Also realize that many fad diets are developed by people with no science or health background.

- Rapid weight loss can result in the loss of body water and lean muscle mass, but not fat.
- High protein diets may increase the amount of calcium your body excretes, and therefore place you at higher risk for osteoporosis (the bone thinning disease).
- Diets that are very low in calories may deplete your body of necessary nutrients that it needs to be healthy, including vitamins, minerals, and essential fatty acids.
- You may become apathetic, irritable, depressed, easily distracted, and less mentally alert.

The next time you ponder starting a fad diet, remember that it may be damaging to your health, so think twice about it.

SUPPLEMENTS

If you are a generally healthy person and eat a generally nutritious diet, then you most likely do not need to take a dietary supplement — you can easily obtain all of your necessary vitamins and nutrients from your food. The Vitamin & Mineral Guide on page 29 lists fat-soluble vitamins, water-soluble vitamins, and minerals, along with their main function, Recommended Dietary Reference Intakes (DRI), deficiency and toxicity symptoms, and recommended food sources.

Individuals who may benefit from a dietary supplement include

- Pregnant women (prenatal vitamins)
- Elderly people
- Strict vegetarians
- Habitual dieters
- People with a food allergy (such as lactose intolerance)
- People who take medications that may interfere with the body's use of nutrients
- People recovering from surgery, illness, and burns
- People with AIDS or other wasting illnesses

The Food and Drug Administration (FDA) does not ensure the safety of supplements. Unlike medications, supplements do not require government approval before they are sold, and therefore it is up to the manufacturer of the supplement to decide whether the product is safe and effective.

Another risk associated with dietary supplements is the dosage amount. Toxic overdoses of dietary supplements can easily occur. Therefore, it is important to adhere to the recommended intake. Remember that the higher the dosage, the greater risk of toxicity.

Finally, some dietary supplements interact with over-the-counter and prescription medications, tobacco, caffeine, and some foods.

For more information on supplements, visit the FDA's web site at www.fda.gov/Food/DietarySupplements/default.htm.

BODY WEIGHT VS. BODY FAT PERCENTAGE

It is not unusual when somebody is trying to lose weight to see that their weight on the scale is increasing and not decreasing as time goes on, despite the fact that they are eating properly, exercising, and doing all of the right things.

This happens because the weight on a scale consists of two items:

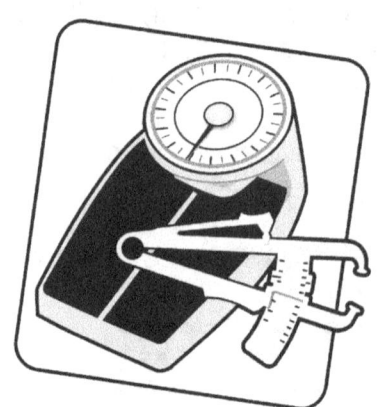

1. Body fat (adipose tissue)
2. Fat-free weight (all of the body's weight excluding fat — muscle, bones, blood, organs, etc.)

Standard scales do not determine what one's body fat percentage is (body fat percentage is the percentage of total body weight that is carried as fat) — just your total weight.

In general, the body fat percentage of a fit individual should be the following:

- Women: 21% - 24%
- Men: 14% - 16%

Therefore, two men or two women could both weigh the same amount and be the same height but have very different body fat percentages (muscle weighs more than fat). A person's body fat percentage can be tested quickly and easily by using a scale that has a body fat feature or body fat calipers. Some people use the Body Mass Index (BMI) charts as a way to determine if they are at a healthy weight. However, the BMI charts are simply a list of suggested weights that show the relationship between a person's height and weight - they do not specify how much of your weight is attributed to body fat or fat-free weight. For this reason, BMI is considered unsuitable for some people, including athletes, pregnant and lactating women, and adults over 65. For instance, a football player may have a very high BMI, placing him in the obese category, but may actually have a very low body fat percentage.

ESTIMATED DAILY CALORIE (ENERGY) NEEDS

As you move around during the day, your body uses energy. Energy in food is measured in calories — it is important that you consume enough calories from food during the day to cover your energy expenditure.

If you consume too many calories, your body stores them as fat, resulting in weight gain. However, if you consume 100 fewer calories per day, you could lose 10 pounds in a year. If you burn 100 extra calories every day by exercising, you could lose up to 20 pounds per year.

Men's basic calorie needs are higher than women's because men usually have more muscle and less body fat than women of the same age and weight. Use the following table to determine your daily estimated calorie (energy) needs.

> "Nutrient-dense" food items contain plentiful amounts of vitamins and minerals and few calories.

- If you are overweight, you may want to decrease the amount of calories that are recommended.
- If you are underweight, you may want to increase the amount of calories that are recommended.

FEMALES			
Age	Sedentary	Moderately Active	Active
18	1800	2000	2400
19-25	2000	2200	2400
26-30	1800	2000	2400
31-50	1800	2000	2200
51-60	1600	1800	2200
61+	1600	1800	2000

MALES			
Age	Sedentary	Moderately Active	Active
18	2400	2800	3200
19-20	2600	2800	3000
21-25	2400	2800	3000
26-35	2400	2600	3000

MALES			
Age	Sedentary	Moderately Active	Active
36-40	2400	2600	2800
41-45	2200	2600	2800
46-55	2200	2400	2800
56-60	2200	2400	2600
61-65	2000	2400	2600
66-75	2000	2200	2600
76+	2000	2200	2400

*Calorie levels are based on the Estimated Energy Requirements (EER) and activity levels from the Institute of Medicine Dietary Reference Intakes Macronutrients Report, 2002.

- Sedentary: less than 30 minutes a day of moderate physical activity in addition to daily activities
- Moderately Active: 30 to 60 minutes a day of moderate physical activity in addition to daily activities
- Active: 60 or more minutes a day of moderate physical activity in addition to daily activities

DETERMINING FLUID NEEDS

Water makes up about 60% of the body's weight. If there is a change in the body's water content, the body's weight can also change (this does not affect a person's body fat percentage). Because the body must excrete some water every day to cleanse its fluids, people must consume at least the same amount of water to avoid life-threatening losses, and to maintain water balance (keep the body's water content constant). Note that eating meals that are high in salt can temporarily increase the body's water content.

Under normal conditions, adults need 1-1.5 milliliters of water for each calorie they *use* each day. (1000 milliliters = 1 liter) Therefore, a person who uses approximately 2,000 calories a day needs a daily water intake of about 2-3 liters.

In addition to water and beverages that contain water, almost all foods contain water.

- Most fruit and vegetables contain large quantities of water, some up to 95% of their volume.
- Many meats and cheeses contain at least 50% water.

Food Item	Water Content
Apples	84%
Banana	74%
Blueberries	84%

Food Item	Water Content
Cantaloupe	90%
Carrots	84%
Grapefruit	91%
Lettuce	96%
Peas	76%
Potatoes	79%
Spinach	92%
Strawberries	92%
Watermelon	92%
Zucchini	95%

Beverages that contain alcohol and caffeine have a negative effect on the body's water balance. These beverages are called diuretics and cause water excretion. For example, drinking beer can cause a net fluid loss rather than a fluid gain. Caffeinated soft drinks, coffee, and tea have a lower effect on water balance.

It is important to drink plenty of fluids, such as water or sports drinks, before, during, and after physical activity to avoid becoming dehydrated. The body loses water through sweating — during physical activity, thirst occurs only after fluid stores have been depleted. Sports drinks contain sodium and other electrolytes that can help replace those that are lost during physical activity.

You can monitor your hydration level by checking your urine color. Urine that is dark gold in color indicates dehydration. Urine similar in color to pale lemonade or weak tea is a sign of proper hydration levels. Do not depend on thirst to monitor your hydration level.

READING FOOD LABELS

Food labels can be used in several ways — some people are interested in monitoring their calorie intake, while others might be tracking their sodium intake due to a medical condition. Food labels are also useful for comparing various food products to help determine which one is the best choice for you.

In 2016, the FDA announced new guidelines for nutrition labels in an effort to make it easier for consumers to make better informed food choices. The main differences between the original and new labels include the following:

- Food manufacturers must now specify the actual amount of Vitamin D, calcium, iron, and potassium in the food item, in addition to the % Daily Value that is already listed. On the original labels, nutrient information for Vitamin D and potassium was not required.
- Nutrient information for Vitamins A and C is no longer required.

- The amount of "Added Sugars" in the food item must be included. This includes sugars that are added during the processing of the food item.

Nutrition Facts	
Serving Size 2/3 cup (55g)	
Servings Per Container About 8	
Amount Per Serving	
Calories 230	Calories from Fat 72
	% Daily Value*
Total Fat 8g	**12%**
Saturated Fat 1g	**5%**
Trans Fat 0g	
Cholesterol 0mg	**0%**
Sodium 160mg	**7%**
Total Carbohydrate 37g	**12%**
Dietary Fiber 4g	**16%**
Sugars 1g	
Protein 3g	
Vitamin A	10%
Vitamin C	8%
Calcium	20%
Iron	45%

* Percent Daily Values are based on a 2,000 calorie diet. Your daily value may be higher or lower depending on your calorie needs.

	Calories:	2,000	2,500
Total Fat	Less than	65g	80g
Sat Fat	Less than	20g	25g
Cholesterol	Less than	300mg	300mg
Sodium	Less than	2,400mg	2,400mg
Total Carbohydrate		300g	375g
Dietary Fiber		25g	30g

Original Food Label

Nutrition Facts	
8 servings per container	
Serving size	**2/3 cup (55g)**
Amount per serving	
Calories	**230**
	% Daily Value*
Total Fat 8g	**10%**
Saturated Fat 1g	**5%**
Trans Fat 0g	
Cholesterol 0mg	**0%**
Sodium 160mg	**7%**
Total Carbohydrate 37g	**13%**
Dietary Fiber 4g	**14%**
Total Sugars 12g	
Includes 10g Added Sugars	**20%**
Protein 3g	
Vitamin D 2mcg	10%
Calcium 260mg	20%
Iron 8mg	45%
Potassium 235mg	6%

* The % Daily Value (DV) tells you how much a nutrient in a serving of food contributes to a daily diet. 2,000 calories a day is used for general nutrition advice.

New Food Label

Serving Size/Servings Per Container

The calorie and nutrient information listed on food labels is based on a single serving size. Therefore, it is important to understand what the serving size is for a particular food item. For example, if two serving sizes are being consumed in a meal, then it is necessary to double the stated calories and nutrient information on the food label to determine what your actual intake is.

When comparing products, check to make sure that the serving sizes are comparable. Food labels also display the number of servings that are contained in the entire package.

There is much confusion over the terms *serving sizes* and *portion sizes*. What is the difference?

- Serving size — the amount of food recommended by the USDA
- Portion size — the amount of a food you choose to eat at any one time, which may be more or less than a serving

To determine how good you are at determining proper portion sizes, try this experiment at home: without using a measuring cup, pour what you think is one cup of dry cereal into a bowl, or one cup of milk into a glass. Now check the actual amounts with a measuring cup. How accurate were you?

Calories/Calories from Fat

> Calorie Values:
>
> Fat: 9 cal/gram
> Carbs: 4 cal/gram
> Protein: 4 cal/gram
> Alcohol: 7 cal/gram

The total number of calories (energy)/calories (energy) from fat per serving. This helps you determine if the food item is high or low in total fat — if most of the calories in the food item come from fat, then the food item is high in fat, and vice versa.

Total Fat

The total amount (grams) of all fat in a serving. The breakdown shows the total amount of saturated fat, trans fat, polyunsaturated fat, and monounsaturated fat per serving size. Choose foods that contain low amounts of saturated and trans fat, and replace them with foods containing unsaturated fat.

Saturated Fat

Saturated fat occurs naturally in food and is normally solid at room temperature. Food items that contain saturated fat are also high in cholesterol, therefore raising your cholesterol levels and placing you at increased risk for heart disease and stroke. Food items that tend to be high in saturated fat include meat and dairy products, baked goods, and fried foods. Limit your saturated fat intake to seven percent of the total calories you consume in a day.

Trans Fat

Like saturated fat, trans fat tends to raise your cholesterol levels, which in turn increases your risk of heart disease. Trans fat also lowers your good (HDL) cholesterol levels. Trans fat is produced when a food manufacturer takes a vegetable oil and adds hydrogen to it. In other words, liquid oil is made into solid fat, like shortening and hard margarine/butter. This process, called hydrogenation, increases the shelf life and the flavor stability of food containing these ingredients. Trans fats tend to be found in food items such as crackers, candy, cookies, and fried foods.

The FDA requires that food labels contain the amount of trans fat in each serving, unless it is less than 0.5 grams per serving. Therefore, it is important to read the ingredients on the label to see if the food item really does contain trans fat. The ingredient list will reference shortening or partially hydrogenated vegetable oil. Limit your trans fat intake to one percent of the total calories you consume in a day.

Polyunsaturated Fat

Polyunsaturated fats are typically liquid at room temperature and when they are chilled. They can help reduce bad cholesterol (LDL) levels in your blood, therefore decreasing your risk of heart disease and stroke, if they are consumed in moderation and when used to replace saturated fats or trans fats.

Polyunsaturated fats also contain essential fats (fats that your body needs but can't produce itself – they must be obtained through food), such as omega-6 and omega-3. Food items high in polyunsaturated fat include vegetable oils (i.e. soybean oil, corn oil, and safflower oil), fatty fish (i.e. salmon, mackerel, herring, and trout), and various nuts and seeds (i.e. walnuts and sunflower seeds).

Monounsaturated Fat

Monounsaturated fats are typically liquid at room temperature but start to turn solid when chilled. They can help reduce bad cholesterol (LDL) levels in your blood, therefore decreasing your risk of heart disease and stroke, if they are consumed in moderation and when used to replace saturated fats or trans fats.

Monounsaturated fats also provide nutrients to help develop and maintain your body's cells, and are high in vitamin E. Food items high in monounsaturated fat include vegetable oils (i.e. olive, canola, peanut, sunflower, and sesame oils), avocados, peanut butter, and various nuts and seeds.

Cholesterol

The total amount (milligrams) of cholesterol per serving. Choose foods that are low in cholesterol.

Cholesterol is a soft, fat-like substance that is made in the liver and found in certain foods, such as meat, eggs, and dairy products. The body needs cholesterol to function properly — the body's cell walls (membranes) need cholesterol in order to produce hormones, vitamin D, and the bile acids that help to digest fat. However, the body only requires a small amount of cholesterol — too much cholesterol can lead to an increased risk of heart disease and stroke.

When there is too much cholesterol in the body, plaque (a thick, hard deposit) can form in the body's arteries, thereby narrowing the amount of room for blood to flow to the heart. Over time, this buildup causes atherosclerosis (hardening of the arteries), which can lead to heart disease. The arteries that feed the heart can become so clogged that the blood flow is reduced, causing chest pain (angina). If a blood clot forms and blocks the artery, a heart attack can occur. Likewise, if a blood clot blocks an artery leading to or in the brain, a stroke can occur.

Types of Cholesterol

There are two types of cholesterol:

- HDL (high-density lipoprotein) — HDL is considered to be the "good" cholesterol. This type of cholesterol carries harmful cholesterol away from the arteries and helps protect from heart attack and stroke. Therefore, the higher your HDL cholesterol, the better.
- LDL (low-density lipoprotein) — LDL is considered to be the "bad" cholesterol. It is the main carrier of harmful cholesterol in your blood. When there is too much LDL cholesterol in your blood, it can join with fats and other substances to build up in the inner walls of your arteries,

increasing the risk of heart attack and stroke. Therefore, the lower your LDL cholesterol, the better.

Cholesterol Levels

A blood test must be performed to determine what your cholesterol levels are. The test will provide you with your Total Cholesterol, HDL cholesterol, and LDL cholesterol levels.

Total Cholesterol

- Less than 200 mg/dL = Desirable
- 200 to 239 mg/dL = Borderline high cholesterol
- 240 mg/dL and above = High blood cholesterol

HDL Cholesterol

- Less than 40 mg/dL (men) = Low HDL
- Less than 50 mg/dL (women) = Low HDL
- 40 to 59 mg/dL = Borderline HDL
- 60 mg/dL and above = High HDL

LDL Cholesterol

- Less than 70 mg/dL = Optional goal if you are at very high risk of a heart attack or death from heart attack
- Less than 100 mg/dL = Optimal goal
- 100 to 129 mg/dL = Above optimal
- 130 to 159 mg/dL = Borderline high LDL
- 160 to 189 mg/dL = High LDL
- 190 mg/dL and above = Very high LDL

Lowering LDL Cholesterol

There are many things that can be done to help lower LDL cholesterol, including the following:

- Engage in physical activity at least 30 minutes on most or all days of the week.
- Lose weight if necessary.
- Consume food that is low in saturated fat and cholesterol, and high in fiber. Decrease foods that are high in saturated fat and cholesterol.

What to Eat

- A variety of fruits and vegetables
- A variety of grain products (such as bread, cereal, rice and pasta, whole grains)
- Fat-free and low-fat milk products
- Lean meats and poultry without skin
- Fatty fish (baked or grilled)
- Beans and peas
- Nuts and seeds in limited amounts (four to five servings per week)

- Unsaturated vegetable oils, such as canola, corn, olive, safflower, and soybean oils (only consume a limited amount of margarines and spreads made from them)

Foods to Limit

- Whole milk, cream, and ice cream
- Butter, egg yolks, and cheese (including foods made with them)
- Organ meats (such as liver, kidney, and brain)
- High-fat, processed meats (such as sausage, bologna, salami, and hot dogs)
- Fatty meats that aren't trimmed
- Duck and goose meat (raised for market)
- Bakery goods made with egg yolks and saturated fats
- Saturated oils (such as coconut oil, palm oil, and palm kernel oil)
- Solid fats (such as shortening, partially hydrogenated margarine, and lard)
- Fried foods

Cooking Tips

- When broiling, roasting, or baking, drain off the fat during cooking.
- Don't baste using drippings — use fruit juice or marinade.
- Broil or grill food instead of pan-frying.
- Cut off all visible fat from meat before cooking, and remove all the skin from poultry. (If you are roasting chicken or turkey, remove the skin after cooking.)
- Use a vegetable oil spray to brown or saute foods.
- Make recipes or egg dishes using egg whites or egg substitutes — do not use the yolks.
- Instead of regular cheese, use low-fat cottage cheese, part-skim milk mozzarella, and other fat-free or low-fat cheeses.

Sodium

The total amount (milligrams) of sodium per serving. The American Heart Association recommends limiting sodium consumption to 2300 mg a day.

Salt is a necessity for body regulation, as the sodium that comes from salt regulates the body's heartbeat and balances body fluids. Therefore, both excess sodium and a sodium deficiency can be harmful. Note that few diets lack sodium in them.

Excess Sodium

Most people consume far more sodium (salt) than their bodies need. Excessive sodium can temporarily retain excessive fluids in the body. This can then become a burden on the kidneys, heart, and blood vessels, especially in "salt-sensitive" people.

As a result, the following medical conditions can develop:

- Increased/high blood pressure
- Coronary heart disease
- Stroke
- Congestive heart failure

- Kidney disease

Consuming too much sodium and not enough water can cause dehydration or make it worse. Understand that the body's kidneys only retain the amount of sodium that the body actually needs, and gets rid of the extra sodium through urine and water. This causes water to be wasted, hence the need for more water.

How is Sodium Consumed?

Sodium is consumed by the following:

- Processed food/fast food - 77%
- Occurs naturally through food - 12%
- At the table (salt shaker) - 6%
- During cooking - 5%

Sodium-Restricted Diets

People diagnosed with certain medical conditions are sometimes put on sodium-restricted diets by their doctor, such as a limitation of 2000 mg of sodium per day. According to the American Heart Association, adults generally should not consume more than 2300 mg of sodium per day. The average American consumes 2900 - 4300 mg of sodium per day.

This lifestyle change can be difficult for many people, especially for older adults. Many older adults are accustomed to certain eating habits and either do not want to change them, or see no reason to change them, despite their health condition. Therefore, it is recommended that changing salt intake habits occur gradually over time.

Sodium Content of Food

Following are examples showing the amount of sodium in various food items:

Item	Portion	Sodium
Dill pickle	1	930 mg
Tomato sauce	1 cup	1500 mg
Hot dog	1	1100 mg
Bacon	1 piece	115 mg
Soy sauce	1 tbsp.	1030 mg
Chicken broth	1 cup	960 mg
Salt	1 tsp.	2300 mg

Alternative Names for Sodium

Other names that are used for sodium on food labels include:

- Baking powder
- Baking soda
- Monosodium glutamate
- MSG
- Sea salt
- Sodium chloride
- Sodium nitrate

Nutrient Claims

Nutrient claims on food packaging must be in accordance with strict government regulations:

- Sodium Free — contains less than 5 milligrams sodium per serving than the original food item (usually the same brand)
- Very Low Sodium — contains 35 milligrams of sodium or less per serving than the original food item (usually the same brand)
- Low Sodium — contains 140 milligrams of sodium or less per serving than the original food item (usually the same brand)
- Less/Fewer — has at least 25% less per serving than a similar referenced food
- Reduced — has at least 25% less per serving than the original food item (usually the same brand)

Natural Salt Alternatives

There are numerous salt alternatives that can add flavor to meals.

Spices:

- Allspice
- Caraway
- Cinnamon
- Curry powder
- Dry mustard
- Ginger
- Nutmeg
- Paprika
- Pepper (red or black)

Herbs:

- Basil
- Bay leaves
- Oregano
- Parsley
- Rosemary
- Sage
- Thyme

Onions:

- Chives
- Garlic
- Onions
- Scallions

Citrus:

- Lemon juice
- Lime juice

Lowering Sodium Consumption

- Do not add salt to your food at the table. Do not keep the salt shaker on the table.
- Avoid obviously salty foods. These include pretzels, potato chips, pickles, and salted nuts.
- Be selective when eating out. Ask if food can be prepared without salt. In addition, ask if any sauces, gravies, and dressings can be served on the side.
- Rinse canned foods such as vegetables, beans, and shellfish to reduce the amount of salt.

Total Carbohydrate

The total amount (grams) of carbohydrate per serving, including starch, dietary fiber, and sugars. Carbohydrates are where most of our body's energy comes from, and complex carbohydrates are the preferred source.

- Simple carbohydrates — also known as the "bad carbs." What makes them bad? They are generally low in fiber and other nutrients; consist of empty calories that get converted into fat; and they raise your glucose levels, which in turn makes you feel tired. Examples of simple carbs include desserts, sugary cereals, candy, soda, and refined breads.
- Complex carbohydrates — also known as the "good carbs." What makes them good? Complex carbs are generally high in fiber and other nutrients, help you feel full with less calories, and naturally stimulate your metabolism. Also known as "starchy" foods, complex carbs are the preferred source of glucose for our bodies (glucose from carbohydrates is the preferred source of fuel for most bodily functions). Examples of complex carbs include whole grain breads, bran cereal, brown rice, potatoes, and fruit.

Dietary Fiber

Dietary fiber is naturally present in all plant foods, including fruits, vegetables, whole grains, and legumes. Our bodies are not able to digest or absorb fiber — fiber simply passes through our bodies. Diets that are high in fiber help you feel full faster and longer.

Types of fiber:

- **Soluble fiber** can be dissolved in water and forms a gel-like substance. It can help lower blood cholesterol and glucose levels. Soluble fiber is found in oats, peas, beans, apples, citrus fruits, carrots, and barley.
- **Insoluble fiber** cannot be dissolved in water. It assists with the movement of material through our digestive system and increases stool bulk. Insoluble fiber is found in whole wheat flour, wheat bran, nuts, and many vegetables.

Sugars

Sugars include those that occur naturally in food and those added during food processing.

Protein

The total amount (grams) of protein per serving. When making protein choices, choose food items that are lean or low in fat. Protein is found in meat, poultry, fish and seafood, dairy products, beans and legumes, tofu, nuts, and some vegetables.

% Daily Value

The Percent Daily Value information is based on a meal plan of 2,000 calories per day. This information can be used to help determine if a food item is high or low for a particular nutrient. As a guide, 5% or less is considered low, and 20% or more is considered high.

CALCIUM AND HEALTHY LIVING

Calcium is the most abundant mineral in the body, although it is only 1.5%-2% of the body's weight. Almost 99% of the body's calcium is stored in the bones and teeth. National surveys show that Americans do not consume enough calcium.

Calcium is very important in preventing osteoporosis, a disease in which bones become more fragile and more likely to break. It is estimated that 10 million Americans over the age of 50 have osteoporosis, and 34 million have low bone mass. If children do not consume enough calcium during their growing years, it may prevent them from achieving their peak bone mass.

Calcium also has the following health benefits:

- Helps maintain a normal heartbeat
- Helps regulate blood pressure — Studies show that consuming low-fat foods, including fruit, vegetables, and low-fat dairy products, can lower blood pressure.
- Helps the nervous system function properly — Blood needs calcium in order to clot, and nerve cells need calcium to transmit signals.
- Assists in weight management — Researchers have found that if adults consume 3-4 servings of dairy foods on a daily basis, they could lose more weight and body fat.
- Can help prevent colon cancer — Calcium may slow down the growth of cells that lead to colon cancer.
- Assists with muscle contraction — The flow of calcium ions inside muscle cells causes muscles to contract and relax. When exercising, muscle fatigue can be caused by the impaired activity of calcium in the muscle cells.

Note that too much calcium can cause constipation, urinary tract stones, kidney dysfunction, and interference with absorption of other minerals.

Sources of Calcium

The following food items are the best sources of calcium:

- Non-fat/low-fat dairy products (such as milk, soy milk, yogurt, and cheese)
- Leafy vegetables (such as broccoli, greens, Chinese cabbage, and kale)
- Canned salmon with bones, sardines, and shellfish
- Almonds and Brazil nuts
- Calcium-fortified foods (such as fruit juices, cereals, breads, and soy products)

Notice that if you are a vegetarian and do not consume dairy products, or you are lactose-intolerant, it is possible to obtain your minimum daily calcium requirements from foods other than dairy products. You may also want to consider taking a calcium supplement.

Calcium Content of Food

To determine how much calcium is in a food item, read the food label.

Following are some examples:

Item	Portion	Calcium
Milk (low-fat)	1 cup	290 mg
Soy milk (plain)	1 cup	300 mg
Broccoli (cooked)	1 cup	65 mg
Yogurt (low-fat fruit)	4 oz.	172 mg
Spinach (fresh boiled)	1/2 cup	125 mg
Almonds (dry roasted)	1 oz.	75 mg
Salmon (canned, bones)	4 oz.	240 mg
Cottage cheese (low-fat)	4 oz.	80 mg
Cheddar cheese	1 cubic inch	125 mg

THE SCOOP ON SUGAR SUBSTITUTES

Many of us love sweets, and they can often be difficult to resist! Unfortunately, sweet foods tend to be fattening and unhealthy, especially for those who need to monitor their blood sugar levels. Thanks to sugar substitutes, many sweets are now less "dangerous" to consume.

Some foods, such as fruit, are naturally sweet and therefore do not need to have additional sweeteners added to them to make them tasty.

Many food items, specifically processed foods, are commonly sweetened with natural sugar sources, also called nutritive or caloric sweeteners, to make them taste more pleasant. Examples of natural sugars are table sugar (sucrose), fructose, honey, brown sugar, molasses, maple syrup, and agave nectar. These types of sugars not only add calories to your meals, but they can also affect blood glucose levels. Natural sugars contain four calories per gram of sugar (1 tsp. of sugar = 16 calories).

Sugar substitutes have grown in popularity over the years for several reasons – they can be useful for weight management, they add taste to food while adding few or no calories, and they help in managing blood glucose levels. Sugar substitutes can also help reduce the risk of dental cavities.

Sugar substitutes are divided into two categories — artificial sweeteners and sugar alcohols.

Artificial Sweeteners (Synthetic Sugar Substitutes)

Artificial sweeteners are regulated by the FDA and must be approved for use. Examples of artificial sweeteners that are currently approved by the FDA include aspartame (i.e., Equal, Nutrasweet), saccharin (i.e., SugarTwin, Sweet 'N Low), acesulfame potassium (i.e., Sunett, Sweet One), sucralose (Splenda), and neotame. Artificial sweeteners contain zero calories and are considered to be very sweet-tasting.

Sugar Alcohols (Natural Sugar Substitutes)

Examples of sugar alcohols include sorbitol, mannitol, and xylitol. They contain approximately two calories per gram. Sugar alcohols come from plant products, such as fruits and berries – the carbohydrate in these plant products is altered through a chemical process. Sugar alcohols do have a side effect – because they are not completely digested and absorbed, some individuals tend to suffer from gastrointestinal distress. They are used in many sugar-free products and energy bars.

NUTRIENT CLAIMS

When going grocery shopping and making your food selections, it can be very confusing reading all of the information on the food packages, and in turn trying to make the proper choices. The Food and Drug Administration (FDA) has strict guidelines for food manufacturers on how nutrient claims can be used on food labels and packaging.

Some of the most common nutrient claims seen on food packages are as follows:

- Calorie Free — contains less than 5 calories per serving
- Fat Free/Sugar Free — contains less than 1/2 gram of fat or sugar per serving
- Good Source of — provides at least 10% of the Daily Value of a particular vitamin or nutrient per serving
- High Fiber — contains 5 or more grams of fiber per serving
- High in — provides 20% or more of the Daily Value of a specified nutrient per serving
- Low Calorie — contains less than 40 calories per serving
- Low Cholesterol — contains less than 20 mg of cholesterol and 2 gm or less of saturated fat per serving
- Low Sodium — contains less than 140 mg of sodium per serving
- Reduced/Less — contains 25% less of the specified nutrient or calories than the regular product

ORGANIC FOOD FACTS

When you are food shopping, do you ever wonder about the process the food went through to get to where it is now?

If a piece of fruit or a vegetable has polished skin with no spots or signs of insect infestation, it's probably not as pure or wholesome as it looks. In order for these food items to look as perfect as they are, the farmers most likely had to use some type of poison on them. These poisons are pesticides used to kill insects, weeds, fungi (mold), and other living things that might damage the crops, and are often invisible. Pesticides are used to make fruits and vegetables look more attractive. Unfortunately, some insects have become resistant to pesticides.

Many food items are often coated with wax to protect them and make them look shiner, and waxing seals in residual pesticides. Unfortunately, washing a waxed item will not remove any residues that might be on the skin — you have to peel the skin off to get rid of the residue. Some pesticides wash off in the rain or break down into less harmful substances in the sunlight, but many don't. Some pesticides used on crops such as potatoes and peanuts get absorbed by the plant's leaves or roots, and then spread into all of its parts, including those we eat.

> Organic: a product that was produced and handled according to the rules set by the National Organic Program

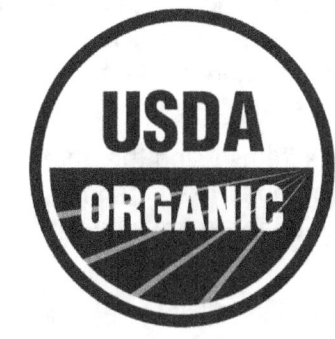

The USDA (United States Dept. of Agriculture) requires that organic produce be grown on soil that has had no prohibited substances (which is most synthetic fertilizers and pesticides) applied to it for three years prior to harvest.

Animals have also been found with pesticides in their bodies. When cows and chickens eat contaminated feed, their milk and eggs can become contaminated as well.

The USDA prohibits the use of antibiotics and growth hormones in organic meat. Organic meat producers must feed their animals organic feed and are not allowed to feed their animals food made from animal parts (this can cause mad cow disease). In addition, organically raised animals must be raised in living conditions that accommodate their natural behavior.

Processed organic foods must be minimally processed without artificial ingredients or preservatives, and can't be irradiated (this is a food safety technique that uses ionizing radiation to kill germs, but this process has been criticized for depleting nutrients and posing health risks).

The National Organic Program enforces the USDA organic regulations, including labeling requirements.

Labeling Requirements

Labeling requirements for organic food are based on the percentage of organic ingredients in a product, according to standards established by the National Organic Program (NOP). These standards apply to all raw, fresh, and processed food products that contain organic agricultural ingredients. Note that organic food cannot be produced using excluded methods, sewage sludge, or ionizing radiation.

- **100 percent organic:** Products with this label must contain only organically produced ingredients and processing aids (excluding water and salt). Products also cannot contain GMOs (genetically modified organisms).
- **Organic:** Products must contain at least 95 percent organically produced ingredients (excluding water and salt). Any remaining ingredients must consist of non-agricultural substances, which are on the approved National List. This includes specific, non-organically produced agricultural products that are not commercially available in organic form.
- **Made with organic ingredients:** Processed products that contain at least 70 percent organic ingredients can use this label. Three of the organic ingredients or food groups can also be listed.

Any foods items using the an organic label must list each organically produced ingredient in the ingredient label. If a person knowingly sells or labels as organic a food product that is not produced and handled in accordance with the National Organic Program's regulations, a civil penalty can be levied.

The term "natural" is unregulated, except for meat and poultry (refers to how meat and poultry is processed, not how they were raised).

> USDA definition of natural: A product containing no artificial ingredient or added color and is only minimally processed. Minimal processing means that the product was processed in a manner that does not fundamentally alter the product.The label must explain the use of the term natural (such as no artificial ingredients; minimally processed.)

What is a GMO?

According to the Non-GMO Project, the non-profit organization responsible for creating the industry standards for non-GMO product verification, a GMO is a "plant, animal, microorganism or other organism whose genetic makeup has been modified using recombinant DNA methods (also called gene splicing), gene modification or transgenic technology. This relatively new science creates unstable combinations of plant, animal, bacterial and viral genes that do not occur in nature or through traditional crossbreeding methods."

Packaged foods that contain ingredients derived from corn, soy, canola, and sugar beet are more likely to contain GMOs. Farmers fields that are non-GMO can become contaminated with GMOs as a result of seeds from neighboring fields drifting to their fields.

HEALTHY SNACKS

Here are some suggestions for quick and easy nutritious snacks:

- Water-packed tuna mixed with fat-free/low-fat mayonnaise on top of whole-grain crackers
- Celery sticks and apple slices with natural peanut butter
- Fruit and cheese kabob
- Raw broccoli and cauliflower florets with low-fat dip/ salad dressing
- Nonfat/low-fat yogurt or cottage cheese with fruit mixed in
- Low-fat/fat-free cheese on whole-grain crackers
- Hard-boiled egg
- Popcorn with light butter/margarine and no salt
- Whole-wheat pita with hummus
- Mini-sandwich: one whole-grain dinner roll with a slice of turkey and low-fat/fat-free cheese
- Mini-pizza: one whole-wheat English muffin with tomato sauce, vegetables, and low-fat/fat-free cheese
- Mini-bagel with low-fat cream cheese
- Nuts/seeds/popcorn

> When grocery shopping, note that the perimeter of the store tends to contain healthier food items, such as fresh produce and meat. The aisles in the middle of the store tend to carry packaged/processed food, which generally contain more fat and sodium.

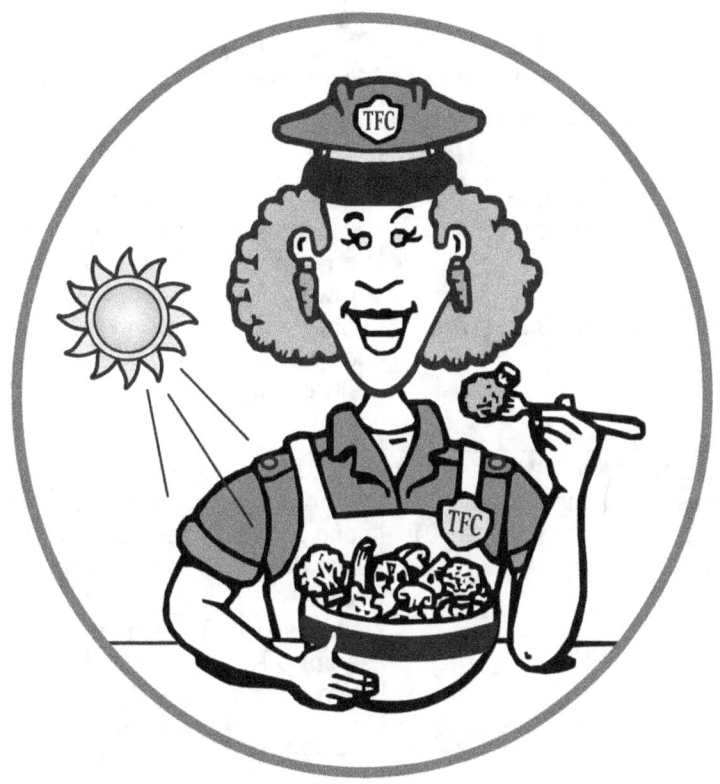

Vitamin & Mineral Guide

This guide contains information about fat-soluble and water-soluble vitamins, minerals, and the recommended food sources for each.

FAT-SOLUBLE VITAMINS

Fat-soluble vitamins are found in the fats and oils of foods and require bile for absorption. Once they are absorbed, these vitamins are stored in the liver and fatty tissues until the body needs them. The body can survive weeks of consuming foods that lack these vitamins, as long as the average amounts provided by the diet over several months approximate the recommended intakes.

Vitamin	Main Function	Recommended Dietary Reference Intakes (DRI)	Deficiency Symptoms	Toxicity Symptoms	Recommended Food Sources
A† (retinol)	Regulates cell growth and cell death. Required for vision. Growth/ maintenance of skin, bones, and teeth.	Men: 900 mcg RAEs Women: 700 mcg RAEs** (age 19 and older)	Night blindness, cessation of bone growth, dry skin, decreased saliva, diarrhea	Headaches, vomiting, double vision, hair loss, liver damage	Carrots (cooked), sweet potatoes, spinach (cooked), beef liver (braised), mangos, apricots, milk
D* (calciferol)	Regulates calcium and phosphorus levels. Required for growth/mainte-nance of bones and teeth.	Men & Women: 15 mcg (age 19-70) 20 mcg (>age 70)	Rickets - retarded bone growth, bone defor-mities, decreased serum calcium, abdom-inal protrusion; Osteomala-cia - soften-ing of bones, reduced serum cal-cium, muscle twitching	Kidney stones, kid-ney dam-age, muscle and bone weakness, excessive bleeding, headache, excessive thirst	Sunlight, salmon, shrimp, fortified milk

Vitamin	Main Function	Recommended Dietary Reference Intakes (DRI)	Deficiency Symptoms	Toxicity Symptoms	Recommended Food Sources
E† (tocopherol)	Antioxidant (protects unsaturated fats, phospholipids, and other fat-soluble substances). Helps prevent oxygen damage in the lungs, skin, eyes, liver, and other organs. Helps maintain red blood cell integrity and nervous system function.	Men & Women: 15 mg	Red blood cell hemolysis, edema, skin lesions	None	Sunflower seeds (shelled), mayonnaise (safflower oil), safflower oil (cooked), canola oil, wheat germ
K* (menadione)	Required in production of thrombin for blood clotting. Involved in bone formation and maintenance.	Men: 120 mcg Women: 90 mcg	Hemorrhaging	None	Cabbage (steamed), spinach (steamed), lettuce, cauliflower (steamed), canola oil, soybeans

† Recommended Dietary Allowance (RDA)

* Adequate Intake (AI)

** RAEs (retinol activity equivalents): 1 RAE = 1 mcg retinol, 12 mcg beta-carotene, 24 mcg alpha-carotene, or 24 mcg beta-cryptoxanthin

WATER-SOLUBLE VITAMINS

Cooking and washing foods with water can filter water-soluble vitamins out of foods. The body absorbs these vitamins easily, and excretes them in the urine easily as well. These vitamins are not stored extensively in tissues, as they are constantly exchanging materials with body fluids.

Vitamin	Main Function	Recommended Dietary Reference Intakes (DRI)	Deficiency Symptoms	Toxicity Symptoms	Recommended Food Sources
B1† (Thiamin)	Part of a coenzyme used in energy metabolism. Supports normal appetite and nervous system function. Required for RNA and DNA synthesis.	Men: 1.2 mg Women: 1.1 mg	Fatigue, muscle weakness, confusion, edema, enlarged heart, heart failure (beriberi)	None	Pork chops, sunflower seeds, enriched cereal, green peas (cooked), baked potatoes, whole-wheat bagels, enriched pasta, black beans (cooked), watermelon
B2† (Riboflavin)	Part of a coenzyme used in energy metabolism. Supports normal vision and skin health.	Men: 1.3 mg Women: 1.1 mg	Dermatitis, glossitis, photophobia	None	Beef liver (braised), enriched cereal, milk, cottage cheese, yogurt (plain), mushrooms (cooked), spinach (cooked)
B3† (Niacin)	Part of a coenzyme used in energy metabolism and synthesis of fatty acids, steroid hormones, and proteins.	Men: 16 mg Women: 14 mg	Dermatitis, diarrhea, dementia, death (pellagra)	Flushing, gastric ulcers, low blood pressure, nausea, vomiting, liver damage, diarrhea	Chicken breast, tuna (in water), pork chops, mushrooms (cooked), baked potatoes, enriched cereal
B6† (Pyridoxine, Pyridoxal, Pyridoxamine)	Part of a coenzyme used in amino acid and fatty acid metabolism. Helps convert tryptophan to niacin and to make red blood cells.	Men: 1.3 mg (age 19- 50) 1.7 mg (>age 51) Women: 1.3 mg (age 19- 50) 1.5 mg (>age 51)	Dermatitis, glossitis, seizures, anemia	Depression, irritability, fatigue, headaches	Beef liver (braised), bananas, chicken breast, baked potatoes, sweet potatoes (cooked), spinach (cooked)

Vitamin	Main Function	Recommended Dietary Reference Intakes (DRI)	Deficiency Symptoms	Toxicity Symptoms	Recommended Food Sources
B12† (cobala- min)	Part of a coen- zyme used in cell synthesis and red blood cell matura- tion. Helps main- tain nerve cells.	Men & Women: 2.4 mcg	Indigestion, diarrhea or constipation, weight loss, macrocytic anemia, fatigue, poor memory, irri- tability, parasthesia of the hands and feet	None	Sirloin steak, tuna (in water), sardines, chicken liver, pork roast (lean), swiss cheese, cottage cheese
C† (ascorbic acid)	Antioxidant needed for colla- gen synthesis (wound healing, blood vessel integ- rity, maintenance of gums, bone growth and main- tenance). Helps iron absorption.	Men: 90 mg Women: 75 mg	Bleeding gums, delayed wound heal- ing, hemor- rhaging, softening of the bones, easy frac- tures (scurvy)	Diarrhea, nausea, headaches, hot flashes, fatigue, insomnia	Orange juice, straw- berries, grapefruit, broccoli (cooked), bok choy (cooked), green pepper (raw), sweet red pepper (raw), brussels sprouts (cooked)
Folate† (folic acid)	Part of a coen- zyme needed for DNA and RNA synthesis, red blood cell matura- tion. Important for reproduction.	Men & Women: 400 mcg (Pregnant women: 600 mcg)	Diarrhea, macrocytic anemia, confusion, depression, fatigue, prevention of birth defects	Masks vita- min B12 defi- ciency	Beef liver (braised), lentils (cooked), pinto beans (cooked), avocado, asparagus, spinach (raw), beets, enriched cereal
Biotin*	A cofactor for sev- eral enzymes used in energy metabo- lism, fat synthe- sis, amino acid metabolism, and glycogen synthe- sis.	Men & Women: 30 mcg	Loss of appe- tite, fatigue, depression, dry skin, heart abnor- malities	None	Cauliflower, liver, pea- nuts, cheese, egg yolks (cooked)

Vitamin	Main Function	Recommended Dietary Reference Intakes (DRI)	Deficiency Symptoms	Toxicity Symptoms	Recommended Food Sources
Choline*	A methyl donor. A component of bile and of neurotransmitter acetylcholine.	Men: 550 mg Women: 425 mg	Liver damage	Body odor, sweating, liver damage, reduced growth rate, low blood pressure, salivation	Milk, liver, egg yolk, peanuts
Pantothenic acid*	Part of a coenzyme used in energy metabolism.	Men & Women: 5 mg	General failure of all body systems	None	Meat, mushrooms, oats

† Recommended Dietary Allowance (RDA)

* Adequate Intake (AI)

**RAEs (retinol activity equivalents): 1 RAE = 1 mcg retinol, 12 mcg beta-carotene, 24 mcg alpha-carotene, or 24 mcg beta-cryptoxanthin

MINERALS

Minerals are needed for the growth and regulation of body processes, including maintaining fluid balance and regulating muscle contraction.

Mineral	Main Function	Recommended Dietary Reference Intakes (DRI)	Deficiency Symptoms	Toxicity Symptoms	Recommended Food Sources
Calcium*	Structural material for bones and teeth. Helps regulate muscle contraction, nerve conduction, regulation of cell activities, blood clotting, blood pressure, and immune defenses.	Men & Women: 1000 mg (<age 50) 1200 mg (>age 50)	Arm and leg numbness, brittle fingernails, heart palpitations, insomnia, muscle cramps, osteoporosis	Kidney stones, impaired absorption of iron	Milk, cheddar cheese, broccoli (cooked), turnip greens (cooked), waffles, sardines (with bones), black-eyed peas (cooked), tofu

Mineral	Main Function	Recommended Dietary Reference Intakes (DRI)	Deficiency Symptoms	Toxicity Symptoms	Recommended Food Sources
Chloride*	Involved in maintaining fluid and electrolyte balance. Part of the hydrochloric acid found in the stomach, which is necessary for proper digestion.	Men & Women: 2.3 g (<age 50) 2.0 g (ages 51-70) 1.8 g (>age 70)	Acid-base imbalance	None	Salt, soy sauce, processed food
Magnesium†	Involved in bone mineralization, building of protein, enzyme action, muscle contraction, transmission of nerve function, blood clotting, maintenance of teeth.	Men: 400 mg (ages 19-30) 420 mg (>age 30) Women: 310 mg (ages 19-30) 320 mg (>age 30)	Confusion, nervousness, anxiety, disorientation, irritability, rapid pulse, tremors, muscle control loss, neuromuscular dysfunction	Cardiac rhythm disturbances, low blood pressure, respiratory failure	Soy milk, yogurt (plain), spinach (cooked), bran cereal, oysters (steamed), black beans (cooked), black-eyes peas (cooked), avocado
Phosphorus†	Structural material for bones and teeth. Important in cells' genetic material, cell membranes as phospholipids, energy transfer, and buffering systems.	Men & Women: 700 mg	Loss of appetite, fatigue, irregular breathing, nervous disorders, muscle weakness	None	Milk, cottage cheese, sirloin steak (lean), salmon (canned), navy beans (cooked)
Potassium*	Involved in transmitting nerve impulses, regulating blood pressure, and controlling muscle contractions.	Men & Women: 4.7 g	Muscle weakness, paralysis, loss of appetite, confusion, weak reflexes, slow and irregular heartbeat	Cardiac rhythm disturbances, paralysis	Milk, baked potatoes, lima beans (cooked), fish (baked), bananas, honeydew melon

Mineral	Main Function	Recommended Dietary Reference Intakes (DRI)	Deficiency Symptoms	Toxicity Symptoms	Recommended Food Sources
Sodium*	Involved with regulating body water distribution, blood pressure, acid-base balance, and nerve and muscle function.	Men & Women: 1.5 g (age 19-50) 1.3 g (age 51-70) 1.2 g (>age 51)	Appetite loss, intestinal gas, muscle atrophy, vomiting, weight loss	Edema, elevated blood pressure	Salt, soy sauce, processed food
Chromium*	Associated with insulin, assists in glucose metabolism.	Men: 35 mcg (<age 50) 30 mcg (>age 50) Women: 25 mcg (<age 50) 20 mcg (>age 50)	Glucose intolerance (in diabetic patients)	None	Meat, unrefined grains, vegetable oils
Copper†	Involved with immune function and heart health.	Men & Women: 900 mcg	General weakness, impaired respiration, skin sores, bone disease	Vomiting, diarrhea	Organ meats, seafood, nuts, seeds, whole grains, drinking water
Fluoride*	Helps form bones and teeth, discourages tooth decay.	Men: 4 mg Women: 3 mg	Dental caries	Mottling and pitting of teeth, increased bone density and calcification	Drinking water (if it contains fluoride or is fluoridated), tea, seafood
Iodine†	A component of the thyroid hormones - involved with body temperature, metabolic rate, reproduction, and growth.	Men & Women: 150 mcg	Cold hands and feet, dry hair, irritability, obesity, nervousness, simple goiter	Enlarged thyroid gland	Iodized salt, seafood, bread

Mineral	Main Function	Recommended Dietary Reference Intakes (DRI)	Deficiency Symptoms	Toxicity Symptoms	Recommended Food Sources
Iron†	Component of the protein hemoglobin (which carries oxygen in the blood) and myoglobin (which holds oxygen for muscle use). Required for energy utilization and immune function.	Men: 8 mg Women: 18 mg (<age 50) 8 mg (>age 50)	Brittle nails, constipation, respiratory problems, tongue soreness or inflammation, anemia, pallor, weakness, cold sensitivity, fatigue	Abdominal cramps & pain, nausea, vomiting, hemochromatosis	Swiss chard (cooked), spinach (cooked), enriched cereal, clams (steamed), beef steak (lean), navy beans (cooked)
Manganese*	Works with enzymes that facilitate body processes.	Men: 2.3 mg Women: 1.8 mg	Ataxia, dizziness, hearing loss or disturbance	Severe neuromuscular disturbances	Wheat germ, bran cereal, pineapple, blackberries
Molybdenum†	Functions as part of several metal-containing enzymes.	Men & Women: 45 mcg	None	Headache, dizziness, nausea, heartburn, weakness, vomiting, diarrhea	Peas, beans, organ meats
Selenium†	Assists a group of enzymes that defend against oxidation. Works with vitamin E. Involved in immune function and thyroid metabolism.	Men & Women: 55 mcg	None	Nausea, vomiting, abdominal pain, hair and nail changes, nerve damage, fatigue	Seafood, organ meats, whole grains and vegetables grown on selenium-rich soil

Mineral	Main Function	Recommended Dietary Reference Intakes (DRI)	Deficiency Symptoms	Toxicity Symptoms	Recommended Food Sources
Zinc†	Part of insulin and many enzymes; involved in making genetic material and proteins, immune reactions, transport of vitamin A, taste perception, wound healing, sperm production, and normal fetal development.	Men: 11 mg Women: 8 mg	Delayed sexual maturity, fatigue, taste loss, poor appetite, prolonged wound healing, slowed growth, skin disorders	Anemia, impaired calcium absorption, fever, muscle pain, dizziness	Yogurt (plain), pork chops, enriched cereal, oysters (steamed), crabmeat (steamed), beef steak (lean)

† Recommended Dietary Allowance (RDA)

* Adequate Intake (AI)

**RAEs (retinol activity equivalents): 1 RAE = 1 mcg retinol, 12 mcg beta-carotene, 24 mcg alpha-carotene, or 24 mcg beta-cryptoxanthin

Workbook

Use these workbook pages to keep track of your daily nutrition consumption, including all meals, snacks, and beverages, and the amount of time you spend exercising each day. Make copies of the pages as needed.

(Is there something you want to keep track of that isn't included in the workbook? If so, use the last column to do this.)

Date: _____   Weight: _____   Body Fat %: _____

Meal Time	Food Item/ Amount Consumed	Calories	Protein (grams)	Carbs (grams)	Sat. Fat (grams)	Sodium (mg)	Cholesterol (mg)	Fiber (grams)	
TOTAL:									

I exercised _____ minutes today.

CUT HERE ✂

Date: _____   Weight: _____   Body Fat %: _____

Meal Time	Food Item/ Amount Consumed	Calories	Protein (grams)	Carbs (grams)	Sat. Fat (grams)	Sodium (mg)	Cholesterol (mg)	Fiber (grams)	
TOTAL:									

I exercised _____ minutes today.

CUT HERE ✂

Date: _____ Weight: _____ Body Fat %: _____

Meal Time	Food Item/ Amount Consumed	Calories	Protein (grams)	Carbs (grams)	Sat. Fat (grams)	Sodium (mg)	Cholesterol (mg)	Fiber (grams)	
TOTAL:									

I exercised _____ minutes today.

CUT HERE ✂

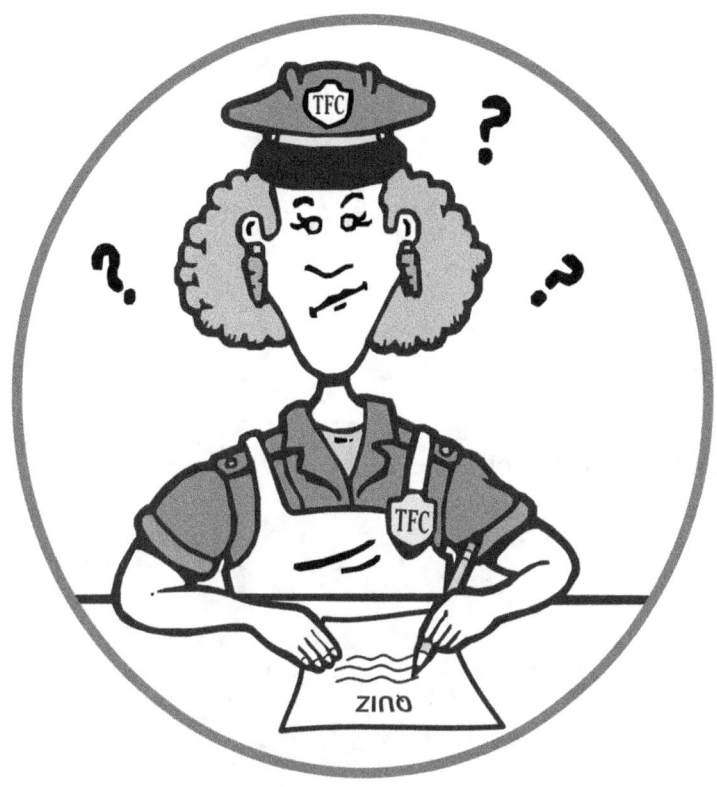

Nutrition Quiz Answers

Here are the answers!
How did you do?

Answers

1. Monounsaturated and polyunsaturated fat
2. High-calorie but good for you in small doses
3. Insufficient nutrients
4. Protein
5. A high-calorie diet
6. Gain weight
7. Chicken breast, tuna, pork tenderloin
8. Determine its appropriate role in the context of all other food choices
9. Starch
10. Green beans
11. Eliminate fats used as seasonings
12. High fat foods
13. Limit intake of processed and fast food
14. LDL cholesterol

www.ingramcontent.com/pod-product-compliance
Lightning Source LLC
Chambersburg PA
CBHW081420280526
45788CB00009B/3167